For my daughter, Caitlin,
my reason to breathe each day.

The Bravest Man

To order additional copies of this book, contact:
Xlibris Corporation
1-888-795-4274
www.Xlibris.com
Orders@Xlibris.com
70837

The Bravest Man

A Families' Journey Through
Pancreatic Cancer

Cathy Sawyer

This book is dedicated to a woman who has always believed in me. She has continually, over the past twenty years, given me the best advice. She always found the bright side in every situation and always did her best to make me see it. She convinced me to write this, insisting that it would help in my healing process. She made me promise that when I was published (she never said "if") and Oprah called me for an interview on her show, she would get to come along (I told you she believed in me). So here it is in writing, Trixie. I promise to take you to see Oprah, if she calls me.

I would also like to thank my family and friends. I never could have gotten through this past year without them. The people I see and speak to every day are my lifeline. I will always be grateful for the daily support they provided. I don't want to hurt anyone's feelings by forgetting a name, but you know who you are.

Last but certainly not least, my daughter Caitlin. I hope that you never forget how much your father loved you. Being your parents was the best thing that ever happened to us. I was born to be your mother. I love you so much.

A very close friend of mine, I call her Trixie (long story), tells me I have a "gift." My "gift" is putting my feelings on paper. Everything I write makes her cry; she has been telling me this for years.

The hospice nurses said I'd know when it would be time. I didn't understand how *I* could possibly know. Wasn't that up to God? I had been trying to keep everyone up to date with phone calls and e-mails. I remember writing a blanket e-mail the day he died. It said how I finally got him into the hospital bed the night before. How he was still fighting with me about getting up. I felt like I was speaking about someone else. How I, at forty-six, couldn't possibly be talking about my dying husband. It felt surreal, but at the same time, part of me wanted it to be over. He suffered so much; he has had so much pain for so many months. Imagine not being able to keep ice cream down. Surviving on water only and having lost about ninety pounds. John was fifty-seven years old when he died, and he looked ninety-seven. Cancer is a horrible disease and takes so much away from you. I hate that poem that reads "*Cancer can't take . . .*" It took my daughter's father away two months before her thirteenth birthday.

It took a brother, friend, uncle, godfather, brother-in-law, son-in-law, and husband on that day. February 14, 2008, Valentine's Day, my husband left his two sweethearts and joined his other sweetheart in heaven; it gives me peace to think of it that way. When he died, I wrote his eulogy to read at the wake. Of course, Trixie my dear friend cried once again.

I went up to the Nortons' place (Trixie's family) for a visit two weeks later, to relax and just breathe. Our goddaughter who is four asked where Uncle John was. "In heaven," I said. "When is he coming back?" she asked. Trixie and I talked long into the night; she convinced me then and there to use my "gift," as she calls, it and write down what I remember of John's journey.

I hope that if anyone is reading this and they are experiencing something similar, these words will help somehow. I hope when I'm done writing this, it will have helped my own healing, as well as my daughter's. I'll start with his eulogy and continue from there.

The Bravest Man

I have never met a braver man than my husband John. His battle was met with a calm and determined attitude. He spent months going in and out of the hospital, went through chemo, radiation, and two surgeries; and yet he remained surprisingly calm. He was always determined not to let the cancer beat him.

John and I have been blessed with the best family and friends anyone could ask for. You will never know how much your phone calls, generosity, thoughts, donations, prepared meals; prayers, cards, and hugs did for us. I will never forget how it felt to be the recipient of such love and kindness. Throughout the rest of my life, whenever I can help a family in need, I will do my best to pay it forward.

I will always be grateful to John for the gift we gave each other, our daughter. He said often that having Caitlin was the best thing he ever did. I remember the day I told him I was pregnant, he cried like a baby. John is now Caitlin's guardian angel; he will watch over her and protect her just like he always planned to.

Right now I have to believe that John is in a better place, where there is no pain, no cancer, and drugs that make you sick. I know that he had comfort in knowing that his mom was waiting for him with open arms. I know that everything happens for a reason. I know now that God took Stephanie when he did to spare her the pain of losing her child. I'm sure when he got to heaven, there was something cooking on the stove for him. It's comforting, knowing that he will be with his mom and dad.

As most of you know, John was an avid fan of the Giants and the Yankees. He got to enjoy the Super Bowl and watch his beloved team beat the pants off New England. So this spring, when Yankee baseball starts, think of John. This fall, when the Giants start to play, remember him. And at Christmas, his favorite holiday, keep him in your prayers. If we think of him often and share stories, we will always have him with us.

When we think of bravery, many times war heroes, firemen, and policeman come to mind. But there's another kind of bravery when we talk of my husband John. He was the one who always got hurt on almost every vacation. He would never take a day off from work, no matter what. So in February of 2007, when he said, "I just can't take the pain anymore" and wanted to go to the hospital, I knew it had to be bad. He spent the next three months in and out of the hospital (mostly in and without a diagnosis) and lost sixty lbs. He had abdominal bypass surgery, then was transferred to another hospital and two days later was diagnosed. I'll never forget that day, May 7, 2007, the doctor said, "You have pancreatic cancer." The first thing John said was, "How do we beat it"?

John and I were married fifteen years at that time. You could say we had our ups and downs throughout our marriage. I even considered divorce once or twice; he probably did too. But our mutual love and parental devotion kept that from happening. Nothing would ever be a greater accomplishment than becoming parents to our daughter, Caitlin.

We had trouble conceiving her. After a few rounds of fertility treatments, I finally got pregnant. Years before I had written a letter to John, I knew exactly how I wanted to break the news to him.

August 18, 1994
To my daddy,

Mommy found out today that I've been growing inside her for a few weeks now. Boy was she excited! She tells me that I'm the most important thing in your lives. Mommy says that you will be just as excited to hear the news. Mommy says that soon, when one of you rubs her belly, I'll be able to feel it. And when you talk to me, I'll enjoy the sound of your voices. Right now all I hear is Mommy's heartbeat. It sounds nice. Well, it sounds like I'll be a very lucky baby. I'll see you in about nine months. You better get some sleep while you can; I like to stay up late.

Love, your unborn child

When she was born, I was thirty-three and John was forty-five years old. We were both married before but had not had children. Finally we were a family and had given each other something we weren't sure would ever happen. I'm not going to paint a pretty picture and say that all was perfect between us after getting this devastating news. But I had never stopped loving him. After he healed from the bypass surgery, he could come home. We prayed he would make it home for Caitlin's confirmation. By the grace of God, we brought him home a week before it. My kitchen counter looked like a drugstore. He was on so many drugs, and still the pain was the biggest problem. They have to kill you with drugs to make you better. She wore my wedding dress for her confirmation day; I had it fitted for her while he was in the hospital. It was a spaghetti-strap straight cocktail dress with a bolero jacket. She was beautiful in it and looked like a young lady. John couldn't believe that his little girl was in my dress. It was a good day; even though he was sixty pounds lighter in his suit, he looked really good. He made it to church (with the help of his closest friend Joe) and went out to lunch with us and actually ate for the first time in months. I remember his mother practically in tears watching him eat that day.

We were frightened that he would somehow hurt himself eating that much. Looking back now, that was the last time John and his mother went out to eat together. He never ate like that again. He started chemo in July. Radiation would follow in August. We worked it out with his doctor so we could schedule chemo around our annual trip to Maine in July. We go with our very close friends, the Nortons—Tom, Trixie, and their four kids (the youngest our goddaughter). The chemo made him tired, but the side effects were minimal. He had a great time in Maine, but he told me he knew he would never be back. I told him to stop being so negative, but I knew he was probably right.

John had a special bond with his mother. She was an exceptional mother-in-law, grandmother, and great-grandmother. She was undergoing treatment for a preleukemic condition called myelodysplasia. When she was diagnosed with this in May 2006, we all thought we would lose her. She spent a lot of time with us and we did our best not to think the worst. The thought of her not being with us was something John couldn't even talk about. Her doctor found a chemo treatment that worked for her; the side effects were minimal.

We had the privilege of enjoying another year with her. It broke her heart when we had to tell her that John had this horrible disease. But like her, we were thrilled to find out that they were to have the same doctor. The doctor found a way to help her; therefore he would help John. At least that was what I explained to our daughter. I wanted to give her hope that she wouldn't lose her dad. But suddenly, after a year of relatively good health, my mother-in-law started to feel sick again. In October, her preleukemia turned into full-blown leukemia. In a matter of five days, she was hospitalized and died in her sleep on October 8, 2007. I had the honor of being at her bedside when she passed. John was at his last chemo treatment when she died. He had wanted to come with me to the hospital that morning, but he knew his mother wouldn't want him to miss a treatment. I had to call him and tell him his mother was gone. My heart was breaking for him. I couldn't even hold him. All I could do was keep repeating how sorry I was. The night of her funeral, John ended up back at the hospital. By this point, everything he was eating he was vomiting almost immediately. He continued to steadily lose weight. We started discussing other places he could try for treatment.

He was not going down without a fight. Over the next few weeks, I would ask him how he was doing over the loss of his mom. He would say he couldn't grieve her death because he knew it would make him physically sick. He knew how that would have made his mom feel. I know how much he missed her; we all did. I wrote a eulogy to read at her wake to summarize the impact she had on other people during her lifetime.

My Mother-in-law

My mother-in-law is an inspiration to us all. As a child, she had nothing, she had no home, no love from a family, and no money. She made a life for herself as soon as she was old enough. Instead of being bitter and angry because of her upbringing, she became a loving, considerate, and thoughtful person. She would give any one of us the shirt off her back or the last dollar in her purse. Her only wish for any of us would be to be happy.

Having only herself for so long, she longed for a family. Boy did she get one, a son and a daughter whom she loved with all she had. She had eleven great-grandchildren. To say she loved them was an understatement; every one of those children made her smile.

We need to take all of our memories and think of her often; doing that will ensure we always honor her. Every time I hear an off-color joke, I'll think of her. Every time I eat a Christmas cookie, I'll think of her (though they'll never be as good). Living our lives the way she did is a wonderful way of honoring HER life.

You always knew she was nearby because you heard her laughing somewhere. She would hate the thought of all of us sitting around crying. So think of a great memory, hold it in your heart, and share it with your children. In this way, we will ALWAYS have her with us.

Thanksgiving, and John is still in the hospital and it is our very first holiday without his mother. Depressing is putting it mildly; we were supposed to be all together.

John was unable to eat anything; he was on a feeding bag. He could take nothing by mouth, not even his medication.

He was going to spend Thanksgiving in the hospital. The only saving grace was an antianxiety drug they had him on that made him sleep a lot. He slept through the day. We ate dinner with our dear friends, Andrea and Joe. My mom, Caitlin, and I could not bear to eat at home. Joe and John had been friends for about thirty years. Andrea and I met through them. She is like a sister to me, we share a lot. I cannot tell you how many hours I have spent on the phone with her crying and ranting. She was never too tired or busy for me. Andrea always let me say whatever I needed to. She made jokes, said inspirational words, and cried with me. She has been a savior like so many others in my life. I have been blessed with a great network of friends. I am truly blessed by that.

He needed another bypass surgery, this time in the intestines. Radiation was to blame for this. It caused scar tissue; they said this was why he was vomiting everything up. The passage for food was so incredibly narrow.

Christmas was approaching; Caitlin and I were reluctant about decorating. Neither of us had the Christmas spirit at all. I remember going to pick him up about three weeks before. He was all checked out, discharge papers in hand. As we were about to leave, he vomited blood. "Oh my god, now what?" His doctor said it would be safe to go home, but if it happens again, he needed to come back. I felt like a kid being cheated out of a promise. I remember crying while John just sat there in disbelief. We questioned, "What should we do, stay or go?" We decided to go home; we both knew he would be back before morning. On the way home, he vomited again. He was greeted by wags and *woofs* (Bear and Sasha, our four-legged babies), Caitlin, and my mom. He took a nap in his recliner covered in blankets next to a roaring fire. He had been dreaming about that for weeks. When he awoke two hours later, he vomited again and I called the ambulance. He was home for four hours in all. In the ER, he vomited a few more times; by then he had lost about one liter of blood, they said. Turned out the blood thinners he was on caused the clot at the incision site inside his intestines to bleed out. They reversed the blood thinner, and it stopped finally. He told me later on that he thought he was going to die that night. John actually made it home for Christmas.

Before he left, the doctor said that the tumor was dormant. I explained to Caitlin that it was like a sleeping volcano. That someday the volcano would wake and erupt, but I hoped not for a year or two. We finished the tree and counted our blessings. There was still an arsenal of medication on the kitchen counter. (Prior to this medicine regimen, I could barely get him to take an antibiotic.) But still, the pain was always the issue. He would double up sometimes; it was the only thing that seemed to help. But what always surprised me was he never got angry. I guess I got angry and complained enough for both of us. It was so unfair; he had lost more weight and hardly ate enough to feed a two-year-old. The day before Christmas, my mom drove him everywhere he wanted to go so he could shop for Caitlin and me. He loved to shop and got a real kick out of picking stuff out for us. John looked so frail by Christmas morning, but he was with us and that was what I wished for.

One of the things that I loved about John was the way he loved my mom. He loved her very much and I know how important that is. Funny thing about John I'm not sure anybody ever noticed besides my mom and me, but he never called her mom.

His mother was the only woman who would have that honor. Not that he didn't respect my mom as his mother-in-law; he just couldn't call anyone else mom. He would do anything for my mother. He has comforted her, defended her, and loved her simply because she was my mom. We used to laugh at the fact that John and my mother were closer in age (nine years) than John and I (eleven years).

My birthday is four days after Christmas, and we drove up to the Nortons' place. John drove—he was feeling pretty good. We had a great time. We spent New Year's Eve with Joe, Andrea, and their children, our nephew, and goddaughter. I remember saying good riddance to 2007 and welcoming 2008. His spirits were good; we looked at this time as "his quality-of-life period." I knew the cancer would take his life someday. That the volcano would erupt and we would have to face that. But not yet, not now. That quality of life they promised only lasted about a month. Middle of January, John was back in the hospital with severe pain. This pain was the worst ever. I had never seen him in such agony; he looked like a wild animal. January 16, 2008, I got the phone call that would change our lives forever.

"I have to talk to you, . . . my life is over, I'm done," were John's words. I yelled at him, and asked, "Why would you say that?" I sat with the doctor the next day. The cancer started growing like wildfire and it's in the lymph nodes were all I heard. He didn't give him more than a month or two. How was I going I tell my daughter that her dad was going to leave us even before her thirteenth birthday? How? Devastation and overwhelming sadness were all that we had left. But still, John said, "Maybe I could get lucky and we could find a cure." I'll never forget the expression on his face when he said that. "Maybe we could go to one of those other hospitals where they specialize in cancer." He said he wanted to try. I never took his hope away; I said I would take him to the moon if it would help. I would do anything he wanted.

The next morning I sat with Caitlin and told her everything the doctor said. I will never forget the expression on her face as long as I live. It hurt so much to say those words to her. She sat silently, crying for a while. We cried together. We talked. We cried some more.

He was coming home with hospice care as soon as he was well enough. The nurses said he shouldn't be alone; I would need to take a leave of absence from work. The schedule I was trying to keep was impossible. I went to the hospital first thing in the morning, then to work, home, and back to the hospital at night with Caitlin. I needed to spend as much time with him as possible. I wanted to give Caitlin the same opportunity. Her school was more than accommodating. They offered home tutoring for six weeks. My job as a teacher assistant at an elementary school was extremely supportive. Before I left, they took up a collection of food and money to help me through. I work with children with autism and there are nine of us in one room, the most amazing women I have ever known. God put the nine of us together for a reason. They were and still are my support group. I needed to be with my husband, but I needed to be with them too. How would I ever get through the day without them? During the next two weeks, he needed more surgery. His liver was failing and he was yellow. They attached a bag that hung from a tube outside of his body to collect the fluid that the liver was supposed to drain. The hospice nurses took care of everything. A pain-management nurse set him up with an intravenous pump of pain meds.

He would get a continuous flow every hour. Finally, John would be pain free for the first time in close to a year. The hospice team was wonderful. The nurses said he wouldn't have more than a month. I hoped they were wrong. John was still talking about going to another facility when he felt stronger. I wanted him to hold onto hope; I knew better though. I had read all the statistics on pancreatic cancer when he first was diagnosed. Six to nine months from diagnosis was what I read.

They delivered all kinds of equipment to our house. It now looked like a hospital ward. All of the medications on the kitchen counter were gone except for three. Keeping him comfortable and pain free was now the goal. John came home February 1, 2008. He ate nothing and drank small sips of water. He got around OK; he was able to walk on his own. He chose to sleep in our bed instead of the hospital bed. Who could blame him? He had had enough of that. The pain was being managed; it was wonderful to hear him say, "I have no pain." I hoped that maybe we would get closer to two months with him. Caitlin was happy to spend time with her father out of the hospital. For now, things were good.

John was an avid shopper, to say the least. He made lists every week of all the sales from the circulars. During most of John's hospital stay over the past several months, I brought him the circulars every week. He continued to make his lists from the hospital. He always knew who had what on sale and how much it was. For the first time, he had no interest in those circulars at all. He didn't ask about them or the newspaper. John no longer cared about daily trivial thoughts; he was no longer the John I knew. I didn't really realize that had occurred until I started writing; how sad.

I tried to get him to write things down for Caitlin. I knew she would want to know what he would have said to her at her sweet sixteen, high school graduation, her wedding day. John always had a hard time expressing himself. He said writing such powerful words were too final; he wanted to wait.

I was given a book to read about what the dying need. It is very important to give the dying permission to go. Caitlin and I told John that we loved him, that he put up a great fight, but it was OK to go.

"I'm not going anywhere" was all we heard. Even now, he was not going out without a fight. But that was John; how could we expect anything else from him? He asked the hospice nurse one day if she thought it was worth going to another hospital. She said all the right things, gave him words of encouragement, and told him the truth. I added that he had done everything he could have done already; the decision not to go to another facility shouldn't be the deciding factor in whether or not he did everything he could. I continued to reassure him that we would be OK, that he did everything necessary to make sure of that. I told him that he was a great husband, father, and son. His mom was waiting for him, and when he was ready, he needed to go. We said these things to him every day. And every day he said he wasn't going anywhere.

February 3, two days later, was the Super Bowl. John loved the Giants. Super Bowl Sunday was big. The original plan was to go up to the Nortons if the Giants made it. But that was not possible, so they came to us. Caitlin and their kids decorated the entire living room with homemade posters and garland. Caitlin and I never took the time to watch football before with him; this time we wouldn't have wanted to be anywhere else.

The Giants won, and they did it for John. Everyone that knew him prayed that they would win. Even the die-hard Jet fans in our family. John enjoyed the game and kids, but he wasn't like the John of years ago. There was no screaming and cursing at the TV. He just had a small smile on his face when I asked him if he was happy.

The next day, something was different, I called the hospice nurse to come. John had transitioned. Oh god, what did that mean? It was the next stage of his illness. The nurse said he would be weaker now and more tired. I remember saying to her how I wasn't ready yet. *How I wasn't ready?* Nobody is ever ready for this, for death. I cried a lot over that week. I told him I was scared. I believe this was the first time I ever admitted this to him. I was always the strong one in our relationship. If I was scared about something, oh boy, it had to be serious. But still he said not to worry, he wasn't going anywhere. John was still able to get around on his own, but now I followed close behind. I was afraid he would fall.

His niece was coming from Arizona to visit him. She was his eldest and closest niece. She arrived on the tenth, and unfortunately, he transitioned again that day. He knew she was there, but he was so far away. He stared a lot now; I wondered where he was in his mind. What was he thinking about? He slept with his eyes open. They were so distant and lifeless. He was becoming delusional; it seemed like he was dreaming wide awake.

His comments made no sense and were like broken fragments of a sentence that only made sense to him. I couldn't leave him for a second now; he was so restless. He couldn't decide where he wanted to be; back and forth from the bedroom to the living room and bathroom. I tried to keep him from wandering; he would get so agitated with me. He even tried to hit me a few times. I'm glad he didn't know what he was doing. The nurses came more often; they said it would probably be less than a week. Between my daughter's tutors, the aide, the nurses, and the flow of friends and family, it felt like my house had a revolving door. Caitlin and I continued our mantra, giving John permission to die.

It was hard to have conversations with John now. His thoughts were short statements and partial sentences. He tried to write something to Caitlin one day. He turned a lined pad sideways and drew a line in the wrong direction. Then he wrote across his line, he wrote that he loved her more each day. That is all I got from him. I'm sad for Caitlin; I'll just have to tell her what I think he would have liked to tell her. After all, I knew him best.

Wednesday night, the thirteenth, Joe, Andrea, and their kids came over to spend some time with John. Joe knew that it would probably be the last time he saw his friend. He needed to find a way to say good-bye; not being very good about expressing his feelings made it difficult. That afternoon, the nurses had told me not to let him walk alone at all. I was grateful that they were there that evening because John insisted he needed to get to the bathroom. With their help, we made it, but it was painstaking. Their son Joey insisted on helping Uncle John in and out of the bathroom. I think it was his way of being supportive for his father. It was very touching and I felt badly for him and his sister, Roz, our goddaughter. Children have their own way of dealing with death. I had also finally convinced John that he should sleep in the hospital bed.

There I could sleep, knowing he couldn't get up and out of bed. The night before, I slept with my arm wrapped around his so I could feel him move. He fought me with all he had to get up. I was terrified of him falling and ending up back in the hospital. If that were to happen, he would never get out again. I had to keep my promise to do all I could to allow him to die at home, as he wanted. Caitlin and I slept in the living room that night with John. I remember waking during the night and checking on him. He looked so peaceful. I will admit I checked to see if he was breathing, just as I did when Caitlin was a baby.

Thursday, February 14, just before noon I sat at my computer checking my e-mail. There were a few from friends asking how John was doing. I decided to write a blanket e-mail to send to everyone so I didn't have to keep repeating myself.

Hi,

I'm writing a blanket update on John for all, sorry if it sounds so generic. John has transitioned into the next phase of this horrible disease. He is now bed bound; he is too weak to get up.

But he still is fighting like mad to beat this thing. He tries so hard to get up and fights with me about not being able to. He is not aware of this though; he is under heavy drugs to try to keep him less agitated. Everyone who knows John knows he would never go down without a fight. I pray every day for him to have peace with his death.

It hurts so much to see him like this. I knew this would be hard, but I was not prepared for just how hard it is. Thank you everyone for your thoughts and prayers, I do appreciate them so much. The nurses at Good Shepherd say it won't be long now; we should all have a new guardian angel with us very soon.

When John woke up, he tried once again to get out of bed. He was angry about the bars keeping him in. Once again, I tried to explain that I couldn't let him up, he was just too weak. He relaxed again and slept. Around 1:00 p.m., while checking on him, I noticed he had urinated on himself. He had never had an accident like that before. I cleaned him up and changed the sheets; thank God, I used to be a home health aide. Every time I rolled him, I knew I was hurting him. I couldn't help it. He was so thin; I cried and apologized at every touch.

After I made him as comfortable as I could, I gave him a push of pain meds. It was very soon after that, I noticed his breathing changed. *I knew.* Just like they said I would, I knew he would die that day. I called for the nurse to come. I told him for what had to be the thousandth time that it was OK to die. That his mom was waiting for him and he had never been apart from her on this special day. And for the first time in months, he didn't argue with me or have a wise response; he simply nodded. John had finally made peace with his death. Thank God.

His sister Carol, Caitlin, and I stood at his side and held his hands. We told him repeatedly how much we loved him and not to be afraid, it was going to be OK. Ironically, I had scheduled our priest to come and give John last rights on that day. He came around 2:00 p.m. I was thankful for that. Some people blame God for the tragedies in their lives and for what goes on in the world. One of Trixie's sisters lost two husbands to tragic deaths. Someone asked, "Why would God do such a thing to her twice?" She responded that "God didn't do this to her, life did it, but God was there to get her through it." When I first heard this story, I didn't process it.

It wasn't until John got so sick that I started to really think about what she said. During our journey, I have come to believe that God didn't give John this horrible disease, but he will be with me and Caitlin to get us through this. Perhaps God had a hand in providing Trixie with just the right thing to say, to convince me to write this.

Shortly after the nurse arrived, she said it would be anytime. She didn't even try to take his blood pressure; she said it wouldn't register. His throat was hard and distended. The same thing had happened to his mom when she was dying. The nurse said his body was atrophying, just another unpleasantry of death. His hands were blue; all of the blood was pooled to the major organs. We tried to keep them warm, but it was no use. She left us then, the three of us standing vigil. I was so grateful that he finally was at peace and I knew he was not in pain. His eyes were cloudy and far away. Could he see heaven and all the people waiting there for him? At 4:36 p.m., John took his last breath while we held his hands. I kept my promise to him; he died at home where he loved to be.

I was not panic-stricken or trying to force breath into him. He didn't struggle or gasp; there was such peace in his death. He just didn't take another breath after the last one, that was all. We continued to talk to him, telling him to find all the people that went before him: his mom, dad, my dad, and an old friend. Caitlin was so strong holding her dad's hand, crying softly. She said in her most grown-up voice that she loved him and that it was OK to go to heaven to be with Gram. I felt sorry for my sister-in-law Carol having lost her mom and brother in four months; how sad for her. It is so strange to feel sadness and relief at the same time. I wanted him to live, but not like this. No man should ever be reduced to what he became.

He was a bag of bones, weighing less than 130 pounds. He had lost over ninety pounds, had absolutely no muscle tone, but he never lost the will to try. He was the "bravest man" I ever knew.

A few of my friends at school (my support group) had made arrangements to come over and sit with me. Unfortunately for them, they walked in practically right after he passed. It helped a lot that they were there.

Edna, whom I'm closest to, stayed around until the funeral parlor came to collect him. Caitlin and I were not allowed to stay where we could see him removed. Edna volunteered to be my eyes to make sure his body was treated with the utmost respect. I'll never forget what she did for me.

I made my long list of painful phone calls. My mom was hit the hardest; she hadn't said good-bye the last time she was out. She was coming that weekend for what she believed would be the final time she saw him. My heart broke for her; in a way, she was reliving my dad's death seven years before. My sister-in-law Carol, my mom, Caitlin, and I went to the funeral home to make all the arrangements. It actually wasn't that difficult; I had expected to feel very emotional over every aspect of the planning. I felt quite proud of myself for not crying over everything, I was trying so hard to hold it together for my daughter. I almost made it out of there without one tear, until I read the poem that would go on his mass cards. Once I read those words, which were perfect in reflecting how we would miss him and why God took him, the tears started to flow.

God saw you were getting tired,
And a cure was not to be,
So he put his arms around you
And whispered, "Come to me."
With tearful eyes we watched you,
And saw you pass away,
Although we loved you dearly,
We could not make you stay.
A golden heart stopped beating,
Hardworking hands at rest.
God broke our hearts to prove to us,
He only takes the best.

Something very funny happened while picking out John's coffin. We have a wood-burning stove. John and I, with much difficulty, built a rock wall to go behind the stove and laid a ceramic floor for under it.

Neither of us had a clue as to what we were doing. Completing this was a great accomplishment for us. The stove was something John wanted very much. He had planned to spend many more nights in front of it. I don't know how many nights he fell asleep in front of the fire while watching his favorite teams on TV. Not only was the stove a blessing in saving us money in heating costs, but it actually got John out of the house on the weekends. He loved acquiring free wood, splitting it (on the mother of all splitters), and then expecting me to stack it. Doing this taught him a thing or two about wood types. One weekend we brought back poplar logs from upstate at the Nortons. Poplar is extremely light and makes good kindling. Well, Caitlin learned this from her dad. So while walking around looking at the coffins and what they were made of, she took notice of the types of wood. The funeral director started informing us about the different grades, from poplar to mahogany, to steel. Well, Caitlin announced, "We can't bury dad in poplar—that's for kindling!" I found that extremely funny and fitting, knowing John. We chose oak, one of his favorite woods; it is strong and sturdy, just like John.

I had decided that John would not be buried in the traditional suit and tie. He hated wearing a suit and tie and especially shoes. He always had trouble with his feet, and shoes really hurt him. So I laid him out in Dockers and his favorite golf shirt. It had a Yankee emblem and had the American flag imprinted on it. He wore white socks and no shoes. I know he would have been comfortable.

Anticipation of what it would be like to see John in the coffin was scary. It had been giving Caitlin nightmares. The first time you see your loved one laid out in a coffin is devastating. John actually looked better than the last time I saw him. Every time I closed my eyes, I saw him dead in that hospital bed in my living room. I was grateful to have a better image of him for the next time I closed my eyes. We got through the wake with a wonderful turnout of family and friends. I was overwhelmed with how many people turned out to pay their respects. One of our closest friends, Bill, flew in from Arizona. He was the best man at our wedding. He will never know how much it meant to me that he was there. Andrea, Trixie, and one of our nieces and nephews had beautiful words to share with everyone.

Then it was my turn. I had prepared something, and I felt honored to read my tribute to him in front of everyone I loved. I wanted them all to know *everything* he went through. My mom had spent the rest of the week with us. I didn't have to do a thing while she was there. She was such a help in many ways; I will always be grateful. My brother had flown in from Las Vegas to be with us. He was a big help to me with all that had to be done around the house. I know my mom was happy to see him; we all missed him so much. The following week, Caitlin and I were alone. Just the two of us, that's how it will be from now on. We had to find our "new normal" life. It would take some time. The phone calls slowed considerably, the packages stopped. But life needed to keep going. The tutors came back, and I had lots to take care of. The calls I had to make seemed endless. Caitlin and I were going to take two more weeks off before going back to school and work. We needed to start our new normal life and get back into a routine. Returning to work, getting back to the kids and my support group were what I needed. Caitlin wouldn't admit it was what she needed, but I think it was. Her friends didn't know what to say. She asked how come her friends don't treat her the way my friends treat me. It is sad, but they will learn with maturity and experience. I hope that she someday has what I have.

Last Thanksgiving, with John's mom gone and John in the hospital, it was impossible for me to cook at my house. Easter Sunday, both John and his mother gone, I couldn't bear it. I didn't decorate—not one bunny, egg, or chick was to be found. I made Caitlin a basket, but there were no eggs to hunt for. John loved filling and hiding eggs for her; I just couldn't do it. We colored eggs at the house of my friend from work, Edna. She also invited us for dinner. We accepted, I was grateful; the new normal, right?

March 17, Saint Patrick's Day. I met John twenty years ago on this day. I was hoping that he would make it for this anniversary. It was a sad day reminiscing about the day we met. I sat at the computer that night to write. I cried a lot, too many feelings not to. It was like having fresh wounds. I hadn't cried that hard since the day he died.

As March turns to April, Caitlin's birthday is approaching. As I prepare for her thirteenth birthday, I'm reminded of her last one. John was in the hospital for her twelfth birthday. She wanted a cell phone more than anything else. John's friend Joe came up with a great plan to surprise her and have John be very much involved.

The day of her birthday, on the way to the hospital, John called what appeared to be my cell (because her new phone was the same model as mine) and I told her to answer it. I had set the answering tune to

"Happy Birthday"; she heard it and smiled. John spoke to her for a few minutes about this and that; she told him we were on our way. Then he said to her, "So how do you like talking on *your* new phone?" "This is my phone, OH MY GOD!" was what we heard next. That evening I had invited some family and friends over for cake. I hated that John wasn't home with us. Just before we sang "Happy Birthday," I called him and put him on speakerphone so he could sing and feel a part of the celebration. We didn't even know he had cancer at that time. Now one year later, he's dead. Today, as I write this entry just three days before her thirteenth birthday, I'm really sad he's not here. I'm preparing to give her a happy birthday, and I'm not sure I can. My schedule keeps us busy all the time, there is just no time to get things done sometimes. John and I wanted to make her thirteenth birthday a special one. We had hoped he would still be here, of course. But not knowing for sure, I pushed John to talk about what he would like to give her. He said he would like to give her a diamond heart pendant.

The heart would represent his eternal love for her and the diamonds would represent the brilliance of her spirit. I found what I believe to be a beautiful representation of his thoughts. I know that having something from John that he wanted her to have will have a special meaning to her. My hope is that every time she wears it, she will think of her father and feel how much he loved her. He loved her so much; my happiness for her birthday is bittersweet. I have been on the verge of tears for days now.

It is the night before her birthday. I am writing an entry in tears. I just finished filling out Caitlin's card. I wrote her, telling her why and how I chose her gift. I know that John would have loved the pendant I chose. I wrapped her other gift and decorated the house with a banner and balloons. We always fought about the balloons for every birthday. I always said he bought too many, and he said there were never enough. It seems so silly now; I truly didn't know how many to get.

The morning of her birthday, I presented Caitlin with the heart pendant and explained how I knew from her dad exactly what to buy.

I told her what he said and what it represented in his mind. She cried and said how sad it was, I cried telling her. I said to her how hard this birthday was for me and much I wanted her to be happy. She absolutely loved her new necklace and has not taken it off since that day. I had friends and family over for cake that night and everything went well. Her cake was good (made to her exact specifications), she got nice gifts, there were enough balloons. But all day she kept saying, "I'm not thirteen yet, not until 6:48 p.m." When I asked her why, she said, "I can say the last time I saw Dad was while I was twelve, when I'm thirteen it will feel like it was last year." She misses her dad; this was the first of many birthdays he will miss.

Almost May, spring is here, and the Yankees are playing baseball. It is so funny, I never cared about the score nor was I interested in watching any of the games. But I find myself paying attention if the newscaster announces the score when it involves the Yankees. I guess I feel like I owe it to him to keep tabs. There have been a few times now that I have thought to yell into the next room to tell John something I heard, and then I remember. Today, however, was the first time that it hit me: he's really gone. Caitlin called me to say she was home from school, like always.

But today something exciting happened; she received an application to apply to the Junior Honor Society. In order to receive such an invitation, you need to have maintained an A average for the first three quarters of the year. I was so proud of her I could do the only thing any mother would do—I cried. My first thought was how proud her father would be of her and how I couldn't wait to tell him. I cried harder. For the first time, I was faced with the reality of him never again being here for things like this. Of course, I had thought about these things, but this time, I felt it. On the way home, she called again to say her report card came and she had gotten straight As. This year (seventh grade) has been so hard on her, and yet she managed to not only get As but also maintain them. Her father is looking down on her with such pride, I know he is. He will always be a part of our lives because he is in our thoughts and hearts; but it's not always going to be good enough. I just really wanted to call him today with her great news.

I feel as though everything I've written tells a tale of sadness. I don't want anyone reading this to think I walk around in a fog of sadness all day; the fact is I know how lucky I am.

I have friends in my life who, although they may have a husband and a father for their children, are a lot less fortunate than I am. I have financial freedom for the first time in my life, my daughter and I are healthy, and we have people in our lives who truly love us. I am sad that John is not here to share our lives and watch his daughter become a woman. Also, I am sad that it was his death that gave us the ability to pay off all my credit cards and have money in the bank. But remember, John and I didn't have the best of marriages. I had never stopped loving him; although I fantasized about divorcing him (often), I never even sought out a lawyer. Part of me feels guilty, because for the most part, I am OK without him on a daily basis. I don't miss the arguing or cleaning up after him; being single has its advantages. For the most part, I feel happy and at peace with my new life. But I do miss him every day. After all, we got married for a reason, we were in love once. I have a lot of great memories.

Well, peace didn't last too long; let me tell you something about myself before we go on. I am a passionate animal lover. I love all animals, but dogs will always have a special place. John and I shared this passion, thank God.

Three years ago, we took out a home equity loan to pay our then one-year-old Sasha to have hip surgery. She had hip and elbow dysphasia. It was either surgery or putting her down, the doctors said. So we did the only thing we could—we went to the bank.

This brings me to the evening of May 5. Caitlin and I went to a store we had never gone to before because it was convenient to where we were. It just so happened to be across the street from the funeral parlor John was laid out in. When we left the store, we noticed people milling around a box. I kept telling myself, "Stay away from the box." So what did we do? We went over to the box. Well there was this tiny little kitten in there. Of course, no one knew where it came from. I couldn't just leave her there. My plan was to drop her off at my vet or something. Well long story short, no one would take her. We brought her home, and one look into those blue eyes and we were hooked. And of course, Caitlin kept saying how we were meant to find her because of where we found her didn't help. So that's how Johnny Angel (Angel for short) came to live with us.

Taking care of her has been interesting. It is like having a baby around the house. We have to feed her every three hours, and she requires a lot of attention. Sasha has decided to adopt her as her puppy. Each lick sends Angel toppling over herself. She is so small her whole body fits in my hand, tail and all. John would have loved the way Sasha has taken to her; he loved that dog so much. We are hoping and praying that Angel does not test positive for any of the feline diseases she can pass to our other cat. It would break our hearts to have to give her away, especially under the circumstances that we found her.

Well, good news: Angel is free of any feline diseases. She is a welcome member into our crazy house of animals; she makes it a total of nine. I must be crazy.

It is hard to believe it has been three months already. I want to go to a psychic. I went to an open forum a few months after my mother-in-law passed. I wanted to hear that she heard everything I had said to her when she was dying. I wanted to know that I made it OK for her to die.

I was not lucky enough to get a reading that night; maybe this time either she or John will come through. I believe in the supernatural and the ability to speak to the other side. I want so much to hear John say that he is OK, that he did hear everything Caitlin, Carol, and I said to him. Mostly I want to know if he is really with his mother again. I want to know that he is at peace.

Andrea's son, Joey, asked me to sponsor him for his confirmation. He wanted to ask John, but he wasn't able to ask him because he was too sick. So he asked me to take his place; I thought that was very sweet. I was honored and accepted. I know John would have wanted me to take his place. He would have been honored to be asked.

John's birthday is May 30; he would have been fifty-eight years old. It fell on a workday; I wished him a happy birthday and thought of him a lot that day. I've been grateful that my regular days are relatively easy to deal with. It is those special days during the year that are hard to swallow, like Father's Day.

I was perfectly fine knowing that it was nearing. Sad for Caitlin, but fine, until the teacher I work with pulled out a Father's Day project for us to work on with the kids. It was like I had absolutely no control over my own emotions. My eyes started to burn and I burst into tears. I couldn't believe how quickly I lost control of myself. So for the actual day, I planned to be out for most of it. I was hoping to distract Caitlin and myself as much as we could. We spent the day out with Andrea and her kids. We went to a festival that we had been too many times with John. But it was OK; we had a relatively painless day.

I had to attend Caitlin's induction ceremony into the Junior Honor Society by myself. That was sad; he would have been so proud of her. I know that he still is, it's just different. She looked so grown up and beautiful, and I know when she looked out into the audience and saw me sitting there, she wished her dad was sitting there too.

I've been doing a lot of home improvements since April. Most of what I've done were things John and I discussed doing when we could afford it.

After I finish something I've been working on, I say aloud, "John, what do you think?" Then I'd tell him, "I wish you were here to enjoy this with me." Then one day I thought to myself, if he were here, we would never have done this particular project, because we wouldn't have spent the money on it. We had different opinions on what was necessary. So now, I just tell him, "Thank you." Because of his hard work and insistence to not cancel our insurance policies, I have the means to do the projects I feel are necessary for my happiness. I have created as very serene, beautiful place in my yard off my new patio. I go out every day first thing in the morning and just sit. I listen to the birds, enjoy my newfound privacy, and best of all, I watch and enjoy the wonderful fountain I bought. It gives me such pleasure to sit there and watch the water falling. I talk to John a lot while I sit there. I share with him how I feel and tell him how he would love it. And I ask him if he's really there with me. I miss him.

School is over and summer vacation is here, thank God. I need this vacation so bad. This will be the first summer that I am not working at all. July is approaching and, with that, our annual trip to Maine with the Nortons.

John knew last year that he would never be back there again with us. I feel that we should let that tradition die with John. Caitlin and the Nortons feel that he would have wanted us to continue the tradition. Caitlin thinks that it will be a comfort reliving the things we did together. Like laughing when we see the sight where he fell off the curb. Yes, he actually fell off a curb; the incident was dubbed "tuck and roll." She thinks he'll be there. I'm not so sure; I have mixed feelings. When I sit outside on my patio in the morning when the world is new and there is peace around me, I talk to John. I ask him to give me a sign that he is cool with us going. I don't want to disappoint her; she always has such a good time there, so off to Maine we go.

If I was looking for a sign that John was OK with this trip, I certainly got one. Let me back up a bit and explain briefly the whole Norton and Kramden history. Tommy and Denise (Trixie) were married one month before we were. At that time, the four of us were living on the same property, just in different houses. Tom, being tall and over six feet, became Ed Norton; and John, a bit shorter and a bit overweight, became Ralph Kramden. With that, the four of us called ourselves the Honeymooners.

Denise (Trixie) has been calling me Alice for so long, her children call me that. When they were little, they would question what my name really was. The Nortons call Caitlin the Kramden kid. Their youngest, our godchild, will only call me Alice. In fact, one day my mom tried to correct her. She very indignantly, hands on hips, said, "Her name is Alice."

On our trip, we stopped for breakfast in Massachusetts. It was the kind of restaurant where they sold lots of local wears. We were looking around, and Trixie yelled out, "Oh my god, look at this!" She was holding up a T-shirt with a picture of Ralph Kramden and a caption that read, "The bus stops here." It was the only one of its kind. What are the odds of that? While driving later on, we saw what appeared to be another sign. A Yankee hat on the shoulder facing us like someone placed it there just for us to see.

During our second day in Maine, I went for a walk by myself on the beach. The water was so cold but felt so good on my bare feet. I looked out at the beautiful vast ocean and thought to myself that only one year ago, John was staring out at the same scene himself. The same ocean water that brushed my feet now had brushed his.

So much change in just one year. I said aloud, "John, I'm here, are you with me, are you standing next to me?" A little later on, Caitlin came walking up to me with a look of astonishment on her face. While walking with one of the kids, she found a white heart-shaped rock next to a messed-up engraved "J" on the sand. I believe very much that there is an afterlife and a way to communicate with our loved ones; you just have to be open to it. I believe that if you are open-minded, you will experience it. There might be a logical explanation for all the things I mentioned, but that's not what I want to believe. After all, the date was July 14, the fifth-month anniversary of John's passing. The symbolism of the heart can't be ignored; remember, he died on Valentine's Day. Caitlin and I saved a small jar and filled it with sand, seashells, and a note.

Dear John,

When Caitlin and I went to Maine this summer, we knew you were there. You gave us so many signs of your presence. It was a comfort to know you were OK with it.

We spoke of you often, remembering funny things that happened each year. You will always be remembered and you'll always be with us in Maine.

Love always, your wife and daughter

We plan to bury it at John's gravesite in the future. At the beginning of the summer, I ordered his headstone. We picked a beautiful black granite stone etched with a beach scene. It was a beautiful representation of the things that John loved.

We enjoyed the rest of the summer, spending lazy days as well as busy ones. Neither of us looking forward to going back to school and work. Right before school started, the headstone was ready. They did a fabulous job on it; it was better than we thought it would be. After it was set, we bought plants and a little fence to decorate it. I don't want anyone to ever be able to say, "When was the last time anyone ever visited that grave?" I plan to have flowers and decorations for every holiday so that it is not such a lonely place to look at.

Over the last few months, I've made a lot of changes. I realize now that I've needed to make those changes. I've spoken to other women like me, widows (I don't like that word), and I have learned that I'm no different than most. I guess it's a stage, part of the process. The changes you make around you help you to cope. For instance, one week after John died, I gutted our bedroom. It never really felt like my room at all. The furniture was John's from his first marriage, and I hated it. It was bulky and ugly and took up so much room in our small bedroom. John also was a pack rat—he saved everything. He used to drive me crazy with the stuff he saved. I know now that I needed to make that bedroom mine. A room of my own, a sanctuary. That is exactly what I did. I didn't eliminate him from the room, not at all; our wedding pictures and the picture poster board we made for the wake are all on the walls. I just needed a place to call my own. That's exactly what I accomplished; it is filled with chosen memories.

I've started to notice that I get very angry for no apparent reason. Everything could be just fine, and then for a reason I can't explain, I'm angry.

One of the women from work, Janet, is a widow of three years. She and I talk often about "widow things." Janet tells me that how I feel is one of the stages of grieving. If I'm going to be angry, I want to own that feeling. I do not want to be angry for an unknown reason. I don't want to be that kind of person or that kind of mom that is pissed at the world. So off to the doctor I go. He agrees that what I'm feeling is perfectly normal for "someone like me." So now, I'm on "happy pills" for a few months. With our first Christmas only a few short months away, I'm going to need them.

End of August, and Janet invites me to card-reading party. A woman she has consulted many times reads your tarot cards. This is, of course, right up my alley. I love this stuff, and I've always wanted to have my cards read. She told me that John was always near me. She knew he died of cancer in the abdominal area. She said a few things to make me believe she knew something. In a few months, I'm going to have them read again.

September, back to work and school. I'm not working with my support group this year. But they are always nearby and only a phone call away. It's OK.

October is approaching and, with that, the first anniversary of my mother-in-law's death. I cannot believe a year has passed; it just doesn't seem possible. I'll go to the cemetery and put down fresh flowers for her. I miss her a lot. She wasn't typical in any way. She was eighty-three when she died and dressed like she was a hip sixty-year-old. She always treated herself to new clothes. She loved purses; she had a lot of them. Her hair was always done, her nails were always polished, and so were her toes. She was quite a character. She used the weirdest phrases, always got the name of a movie backward, and always announced when she had to use the bathroom. God I miss her.

I don't want to, but I have to face that Christmas is approaching. I told my mom to go to Vegas and be with my brother. She hasn't spent a Christmas with him in about fifteen years. I don't want to celebrate this year; no tree, no decorations. I finally convinced her, and she reluctantly booked a trip.

Well, as we know, life is unfair, and sometimes I think we are living in hell and death is our reward. What else could possibly explain why a forty-eight-year-old woman would get bone cancer and leave her husband with their seven-year-old son who has autism?

I have known this family for three years now. I am Michael's teacher in school, and I work with him in his home after school. His parents—Mike and Lori—and I have developed a very pleasant relationship. I babysit for him as well over the summer months. I have come to love Michael very much. His parents have been very good to Caitlin and I; we have grown to love them as well. I love Michael as if he were my own son; there is something very special about him. He has the most beautiful blue eyes, and the way he looks at you when he thinks he has something over on you is indescribable. Lori was told early September that her "not life-threatening" lung cancer was now in her bones and that without chemo, she could die in three months. The chemo would only give her an additional three months; she has opted not to take it. She has sought out a homeopathic treatment plan. I pray every day that it works for her; I cannot imagine what her little boy is going to do without his mother. It is so sad that we can talk about all of this in front of him and it's like we are speaking a foreign language. Although he understands our language, he doesn't know what cancer and dying is.

There's a blessing in that knowledge for his parents. The only thing they will accept from me is my time, so I take Michael on the weekends for a few hours to give them a little peace.

Sunday, September 28, 2008, early afternoon was when I sat down to write the above paragraph, and right after the last word, my phone rang. It was Michael's father, Mike, calling to tell me that his wife died this morning. She fell and hit her head and passed away, just like that. He felt that she was ready; he thought she knew she was not going to be able to fight this cancer. Maybe it's for the best that she doesn't have to face the fact that she would be leaving her son and husband. I find it so ironic that I would choose to write about this particular part of my life and how it pertains to my decisions, today. If the phone hadn't rung, the next paragraph would have read as follows: After learning of Lori's diagnosis, I had realized that life is too uncertain and too short. I, my mom, or even my brother could receive a devastating blow that would change our lives forever. I asked John to give me a sign that it would be OK with him if Caitlin and I went to Vegas for Christmas. Christmas was his favorite holiday, and I feel weird about not being here.

I'm afraid he'll be here looking for us. But everyone says that spirits of our loved ones can find us no matter where we are. Caitlin and I talked about it and we came to the conclusion that if we stay home Christmas Day, we would be miserable. We will probably be miserable Christmas Day in Vegas, but at least we will be surrounded by the people who love us. Life can throw many punches; I would hate to think that this was the last Christmas I could have spent with my mother and brother. I haven't spent Christmas with my brother since 1980. I know that my mother will be so happy for us to all be together. She hated the idea that we would be home by ourselves.

Lori is now in a better place where there is no pain or fear. She is in good company; I know John was there to show her the way. They say everything happens for a reason; well, I wish someone could tell me what the reason is this time. I wish I could understand. Her wake and funeral will be heart wrenching.

I'm going to have John's ring sized to fit my thumb on my left hand. I've been wearing it around my neck hanging from a chain since the day he died.

I remember when I pushed that ring on his finger for the first time. That was almost seventeen years ago this November 27. It was a bit tight and I had to push it to get it on. I remember wanting to wait until I was sure he couldn't still feel or sense in any way what I was doing when I took it off his finger. Some say the last sense to go is hearing, others say it's feeling, who really knows. I just didn't want him to know I was removing it. Taking it off was a lot easier because off all the weight he had lost. His ring had gotten so big on him; he made me put tape on it so it wouldn't fall off. He always wore his ring; he hadn't ever gone a day without it on his finger after I placed it there. I was John's third wife; he wasn't a stranger to marriage. But he was very proud of the fact that we were together nineteen years and married sixteen. So when I wrote the facts I wanted listed in his death notice, I made sure how long we were married was part of it. I remember the funeral coordinator asking if we really needed that in there (I guess she was trying to save me money). I said, "Absolutely, we were both married before and quite proud of those sixteen years." I know that would have made John laugh.

We went up to the Nortons early October to apple pick; it had become an annual tradition.

Last year, John was too sick for us to go. We always had a lot of fun when we went though. John was always money conscious. I remember one time about two years ago. It was the last time we went as a family together. He complained because the farm charged you a dollar for the bag you needed to fill with apples. Then he complained about the cost of the filled bag. Trixie kept telling him, "You're not just paying for the apples, you're paying for the atmosphere." So this time when we went, like everything else, the cost of picking apples went up. I made some kind of comment about it, and of course, we heard from Trixie. "You're not just paying for the apples, you're paying for the atmosphere." We all had to laugh, remembering John. We had fun, and spending time with the kids is always good for both of us.

While we were there, another brainstorm was born. Sometime over the summer, I had a dream about one of the kids in my class. He has autism and is nonverbal. In my dream he was delivering flyers (who can figure dreams out?) in front of my house. I bent down to him and asked him if he remembered me. I don't remember his reply, but it startled me to hear him speak at all. When I questioned him, he said, "I found my words."

So while at the Nortons, I awoke after a dream about Lori (Michael's mom). Trying to go back to sleep, I started thinking about the dream that woke me. In doing so, I thought of my previous dream (I don't know why). That's when it suddenly hit me that I should write a children's book about a boy who has autism who finds his words. I was so excited about the idea as I told Trixie in the morning. Of course, she did as she always does and encouraged me to use my "gift," as she calls it. The only two times I have ever in my life been inspired to write have both been at her house.

I've started writing my children's book, and it is going really well. I had actually written the first page in the car on our way home from their house that weekend. Actually, I should say, I had Caitlin write while I dictated to her. I want her to do all the illustrations—she is a remarkable artist. While typing a few more pages a few days later, I remembered something fascinating. Remember that card reader I went to over the summer? Well, I had asked her about *The Bravest Man* project, wondering if it would ever be published. She said I would have success but that Caitlin would have a part in it. So I thought maybe Caitlin would someday want to add something from her perspective.

I figured, whatever is meant to be will happen. I had no intention on pushing that on her. So what I realized was that the card reader wasn't referring to *The Bravest Man* project; she must have seen this new project in my future. And because Caitlin is going to be the illustrator, that is her part in it. Oh my god, I am so excited about this, I feel like I'm supposed to do this. It wasn't a coincidence that I dreamt of Lori, who has a son with autism, which prompted me to remember my dream of the boy with autism at school. That was supposed to happen, those dreams happened to me for a purpose. I just know it. I will dedicate *I Found My Words* (I love the title, it is so appropriate) to Lori, and a percentage of the profits (jumping the gun a bit, I know) will go toward Autism United, her favorite charity.

Caitlin and I have always had a good relationship, at least I thought so. But it was nice to hear her say it, which she did just recently. We do a lot together, such as scrapping and most recently, kickboxing. Andrea had been trying to get me to go for a long time. I resisted the idea, thinking I would get hurt. Finally, I decided to try it. I really enjoyed it, and you can do it at your own pace.

Caitlin hates to be alone so she would come and watch. I encouraged her to try it as well. So now, we do it together. Andrea's daughter Roz joined too. So now the four of us are there together, two mother-daughter teams. This children's book project is going to be such a wonderful opportunity for Caitlin and I to get even closer. I am so excited to be working alongside her on this. I can't wait to see her interpretation of my words with her illustrations. She is a wonderful daughter, I am so fortunate. When I read to her from these pages, she tells me she loves the way I write. That compliment will never sound sweeter from anyone else in this world (sorry, Trixie).

The front of our house looks pretty, decorated with pumpkins and mums. I like the fall, it is my favorite season. I really don't want to decorate for Halloween this year. Thanksgiving will be here before we know it. We're spending it with Edna and her family this year. Wouldn't you know it; fate can be cruel. Thanksgiving falls on my wedding anniversary, November 27. What are you going to do? I like spending time at Edna's house. Her family is welcoming; Caitlin and I feel comfortable there.

Best is, my mom is always welcome there and she feels comfortable as well. Thanksgiving will be fine and we will have a great time. After all, I have a lot to be thankful for.

I have been trying to be a friend to Mike (Michael's dad). I take Michael as often as I can. We really enjoy spending time with Michael; he is such a sweet little boy. I think he is doing a great job of adjusting to his new life with just his dad. Mike is doing his best, trying to cope with the loss of his wife. I have shared some of my experiences with him in the hopes that I can help. After all, that is why I started this project in the first place. I just want him to know that I understand how he feels, because I really do. What I share with him are not just words pulled out of the dictionary—they are heartfelt and real. His wounds are so fresh that everything he feels is like a pinch of salt.

It's hard to believe that Halloween is almost here. I believe that I'm finished with my children's book project. I am inviting a few friends over to preview it for me, to get some feedback. I really hope they like it. I think it's good.

I borrowed one of those how-to *For Dummies* books from the library. It really offered a lot of information on publishing a children's book.

The book explains that you should have a book-reading with your friends to get their input. I'm very excited and can't wait to read the book to them. I sent an invitation to Edna, Janet, Diana, and Danielle. The invitation was made to sound very mysterious. I am having way too much fun keeping this book-reading a mystery. My friends are dying to know why I've invited them over. Some of their guesses have been very funny. Let's see, "Are you pregnant?" That is a good one; it is not physically possible for that one. Besides, if I had gone out one night and had a one-night stand, they would have had to visit me in the hospital after the heart attack I would have had. Other guesses are, "Are you moving?" "Did you meet someone?" I just keep saying, "You'll see," and they keep saying, "It better be worth it." I've chosen these women because the five of us have worked together for the past two years. They understand where I am coming from, and most importantly, they love the children we work with that have autism. Janet especially, because she has a grandson with autism. These four women, I think, are the perfect choice to critique my book. Trixie is equally as excited for her own reasons.

After all, my children's book was conceived at her house, just like this book. I am going to conference call her after I am finished reading *I Found My Words* so she can be a part of the conversation.

Caitlin is running for school president. She worked so hard on her campaign. The posters she made with the help of a good friend are unbelievable. She is very creative, and it shows in her artwork. I know how devastated she will be if she loses. I pray she wins. John would have been so proud of her for even attempting this. This is something neither of us would have ever had the courage to do at her age.

Well, we all have life lessons to learn; Caitlin is no exception. She lost the election. I felt so sad for her. She was devastated, but handled it quite well, I think. There were no tears, just utter confusion as to why the other kid won and not her. Then she said something to make me realize that she too has moments when she misses her dad. Of course, I know that she does, but as her mom, I hope that I've been enough. But she said that in a way she was glad she lost, "Because dad would have loved that I won, and he's not here to see it."

Then we laughed, thinking how he would have gone over to the winner's house with a bat to beat him up if he was here. My husband was always threatening to beat someone up, especially if it involved his daughter. The big bully that he was, all talk, trust me.

One day away until my book reading with the girls from school. I called Trixie to read her my finished work (I hope); she loved how it sounded. I can always count on her for encouragement. She said something really cool. When I was done reading, she said, "Cathy—you found your words." I didn't comment on that phrase, but I did think about it. I have gone through my entire life never knowing what I wanted to be when I grew up. My degree is in liberal arts—can't get much more generic than that. How amazing would it be if, after all of these years, I finally found what I wanted to do with my life? If this book or the children's book ever gets published, I would be an author. I would have not only "found my words" but found myself in these pages of expression. Talk about life changing. Did I need to experience my life lessons before I could figure out what I wanted to be when I grew up? Would I have ever figured this out had I not started this journal?

I always wrote well when trying to express myself in cards and letters. Thank God for papers in college, because that's how I earned my As. But none of that ever made me think I would want to be an author. Well, before I get too far ahead of myself, let's see what the publishers think. Maybe what Trixie and I think is talent is *not*.

Well, my book-reading night was so much fun. Before the girls arrived, I started to wonder if maybe I made too much out of this. I told them I hoped that they wouldn't be disappointed; after all, I had made such a big deal out of it with my mysterious invitation. I explained about my original dream and then about my dream of Lori and how I pieced it together.

When I said the words, "I've written a children's book," the expressions and gasps said it all. They were not disappointed. They took their jobs very seriously; each had a pencil and weren't afraid to use it. They all gave me great suggestions and we did some rewriting. The best was that they thanked me for sharing it with them. I knew I chose well. Since three out of four thought I might be pregnant, we are referring to this project as the "Baby."

Well, I'm finished with the rewrites. My book is ready for the publishers, I think. Today is November 14, and I've just mailed out manila envelopes to nineteen different publishing houses. Now we just wait. I'm very excited about this; it feels so good to me.

Thanksgiving is next week already, hard to believe. I feel settled in my decision to go to Vegas for Christmas. I was really second-guessing my decision. But I think it will be OK, John will be with us, I know he will.

I received my first rejection letter; I know it will not be the last. I know that my children's book will get published, I know it will. The right publisher hasn't read it yet, that's all.

Thanksgiving Day and my wedding anniversary (seventeen years): wow, a lot to deal with in one day. I went to the cemetery alone, and I brought a lawn chair so I could sit awhile. Not too far away, a young woman was kneeling by a recent grave. She was openly sobbing into her hands, it was so sad. I couldn't help but watch her. She looked up toward me and caught my eyes; she mouthed, "I'm sorry."

I responded with the same; for just one moment in time, we were bound together by the same feelings of grief. It was a gift. One of the things I told John that day was that I have been feeling like I might be ready to move on soon. I felt guilty saying it aloud. But he needed to hear it from me and I needed to say it.

If you had asked me in November if I were going to put up a tree or decorate for Christmas, the answer would have been "probably not." Just before Christmas, I don't know when exactly or how, but suddenly the thought of decorating or celebrating Christmas wasn't so sad. Maybe this was to be my gift from God, because suddenly, there was clarity and ease. I knew that *it is OK* to put everything behind me. I will never forget my husband or our life; he will never be replaced. He will always be a part of my past life and always remembered throughout the years. But now is the time for me to start a new life and make new memories and do things for me. Somehow, I just know that it is OK to feel this way, that John will not be mad or disappointed in me. The tree has a lot of new ornaments on it as well as only the special ones from years past.

I bought us a new one, two bears hugging each other, Caitlin and I. We decorated inside and out; we did things a little differently than usual though.

A strange thing happened on the way to Vegas: we never got there. Our flight was canceled, and Mom didn't want to sit for hours or days on end in the airport, waiting for the next available flight. So we did the next best thing—we flew my brother here. Mom was so sad when she realized she would not spend yet another Christmas with her son. When the arrangements worked out and he could come here, she was so excited, the expression on her face was enough for me. We had a great time with my brother here. He is like an oversized child; he gets down on a child's level and has fun with them. So Caitlin had a wonderful time with her Uncle Carl. I think his being here really helped her a lot. Christmas morning, after breakfast and presents, she came to me and said, "Even though Dad wasn't here, Christmas was really great." What more could I possibly want? We enjoyed Christmas, and all the feelings I was expecting to feel really weren't as bad as I thought they would be. We all went to the cemetery that morning. John and I had spent every Christmas together for the past twenty years.

How could I not go to him and wish him a Merry Christmas? It was nice to see that most of the graves in his area were not forgotten. It was like a sea of Christmas blankets.

Andrea had asked me for picture of Caitlin and John, so I gave her one of the two of them on the beach in Maine, the first year we went. For Christmas, she had that picture made into a blanket. It was absolutely perfect. Andrea told her that whenever she wanted, she could wrap herself up in her father. Andrea has always done a great job in choosing Caitlin's gifts, but I think this one would be hard to beat.

My little girl is growing up. A boy at school gave her a Christmas present. She has known Jake (not his real name) since she was in preschool. They have been friends all these years, occasionally being in the same classes. When I got home from work, she looked at me glowingly and said, "Look at what Jake gave me." He gave her a large stuffed lamb from one of her favorite stores. So of course, we had to rush out and find the prefect gift for him. I'm so jealous of that feeling; you never forget those first butterflies.

We'll see where this goes. I'm excited for her. John would have taken this so differently; he dreaded the thought of this day. He didn't want her to grow up at all. Forever his little girl.

Last December while John was in the hospital, there were other families losing loved ones as well. One of the patients' daughters gave me an orchid plant, already in bloom. The bloom lasted for about a month; I continued to water it, not knowing if I would get another flower. In July, when Caitlin and I went to Maine, it bloomed again—two beautiful flowers, again lasting about a month. Well, Christmas morning, two beautiful flowers bloomed again. There are eight others waiting their turn; eight and two is eleven and that is the date Caitlin was born. Nature, coincidence, or John, you tell me.

Four days after Christmas, my birthday, forty-seven today. John felt well enough on this day last year that he drove up to the Nortons so we could celebrate my birthday. That was the last time he drove at all.

Last New Year's Eve, Joe, Andrea, their kids came over to bring in the New Year with us.

It was important for Joe to spend New Year's Eve with his friend; I knew it would be their last. The four of us had brought many a new year together. Although John was supposed to be in his "quality of life" phase, I knew he would probably not be here for this New Year's Eve. I remember saying good riddance to chemo, radiation, pain, vomiting, and empty promises made by doctors. I welcomed 2008 hoping John would have a good part of the year to enjoy with his daughter and some quality of life. Well we know how that turned out. So this New Year's Eve, I said good riddance to 2008 and welcomed in 2009. Of course, I thought of John, but I also wonder what is in store for me, now that I can see me more clearly.

Early January 2009, I can't believe John will be gone a year soon. I'll never be able to let that anniversary go by quietly, because that date is always under my nose. Valentines, Valentines, Valentines—that's all I see and hear about this time of year. There is no escaping it.

Patrick Swayze did an interview with Diane Sawyer recently. He is dying of pancreatic cancer and is fifty-seven years old. His interview was hard to watch.

Almost everything he said that was happening to him was like listening to John tell it. Patrick Swayze even looked like John did last January when John was in his ridiculously short "quality of life" phase. Which leaves me to believe that he doesn't have much time left on this Earth. The reason that this has an effect on me at all is because of a funny memory.

On our very first date, after dinner and talking for what seemed like hours, John finally tried to kiss me. I had gotten up for some reason, and when I returned, John had crooked his finger, motioning for me to come to him. Well, talk about butterflies—I knew I was in trouble. Not too long into our relationship, the movie *Dirty Dancing* came out, starring Patrick Swayze. That movie was quite a hit and popular among the women, including me. In the movie, his character beckons the leading lady to come to him in the exact way that John did it to me. Well, once John saw that, he told everybody how Patrick Swayze stole his move. So over the years, whenever we watched that movie, he always reminded me that he did it first.

When Patrick Swayze dies of this horrible disease, I will cry for that man and weep for his widow.

Super Bowl Sunday is around the corner; what a difference from one year to the next. I couldn't even tell you who is playing this year, since the Giants aren't in it. Had they been, I would have paid attention for John. Last year was so special for John and it feels like yesterday. The last football game he watched, the last sporting event of any kind, the last time he saw the Nortons.

Early February, Caitlin and I are going to Arizona for a few days over February break. We will be there for Valentine's Day. I'm looking forward to the trip very much. I can't wait to see my niece's kids and spend time with all of them. My niece Lisa was the one who flew here to see her uncle the week before he died. She and I were always very close; we are only six years apart in age. She is John's sister's eldest. We have never been to Arizona; I can't wait to see a real cactus.

Finally, it is my turn to inspire Trixie to do something special instead of it always being the other way around. She is starting a writing project of her own because of me. I hope I can help her even half as much as she has helped me.

By the way, still no bites on my book. I have hope that this is going to be my year. Chinese New Year just passed; it is the year of the ox. I was born in the year of the ox, so this is the year that all good things will happen for me. At least that is what Trixie says anyway. I think it was two years ago we went to their house for a weekend just to celebrate the Chinese New Year. It was the year of the pig. We had so much fun. Since January 3, I have lost eighteen pounds, gotten a new haircut, and for the first time in a long time, like what I see in the mirror. I'm starting to feel comfortable in my own skin. I feel emotionally and psychologically healthy. Part of me feels ready to start a new relationship, but not enough to pursue one. I like being on my own. I like where I'm at with Caitlin and our life together. A man would change all of that. Maybe he would change it in a good way, but maybe not. It's not a matter of being "ready" or not; it is whether or not I want to remain "single" at this time. After thinking about it, I really don't want to get involved with anyone right now. I really like being single; it's my choice for now.

We went to the cemetery this weekend to put a heart wreath on John's gravestone. Next weekend is Valentine's Day and will be his first anniversary. Where did the time go?

John is buried in a new section. There have been so many new headstones erected around him. So many hearts broken, dreams crushed, and futures redirected. But life goes on. Every single time I have visited him, there has been a couple visiting a nearby grave as well. The grave belongs to their son, who died at the age of seventeen. Today I noticed that he died 2-14-07: one year before John, but on the same date—Valentine's Day. They sit on lawn chairs, cry, and hold each other. If that doesn't make you appreciate life, what does? The weepiness of months long past is creeping up on me. I feel very sad the last few days. Caitlin tells me that she doesn't remember a lot of the last year. That sometimes for her it still just doesn't feel real. She knows that she's closer to coming to terms with it. Because she had a dream, recently, where she and I were on vacation together and it felt right that it was only the two of us. She has amazing insight into her own mind at just thirteen. I think this week is going to be a lot harder than I thought it would be. There is going to be an anniversary mass held at the chapel later on this month; by then we'll be back from Arizona.

I told my doctor that I don't feel as though I need my happy pills anymore. You have to wean yourself off them very slowly. He gave me a schedule, instructing me on how to do it. I marked my calendar accordingly. Guess what day my very last pill is: Valentine's Day. These things only happen to me.

Caitlin and I made it to Arizona. We had a great time. It was so nice spending time with my niece and her family. Our first full day there was Valentine's Day. Lisa (my niece) was telling her girls that this was the day that Uncle John died. I told the girls that instead of being sad, I wanted them to see it as Uncle John's first anniversary in heaven. I told them, "We should all wish him a happy anniversary." I didn't want them or us to be sad. I set my phone to go off at 4:36 p.m. precisely, signifying John's first anniversary in heaven. When it rang, with a single tear in my eye, we wished John a happy anniversary. Many people remembered what day it was; I received a lot of phone calls and texts. You really know who your friends are and who really loves you on days like that. I am so grateful and feel so lucky. Arizona is a beautiful state, and yes, I did get to see a lot of cactus.

February 21, the cemetery held an anniversary mass. My mom, Joe, Andrea, their kids, my cousins Pat and Charlie and their daughter Zoey were there. We took up about half of the chapel with our little crowd. It meant a lot to me that they were all there. The priest did a beautiful job with the service, we were all very impressed. Afterward, we went over to John's grave. It was the first time that Joe had seen it, as well as my cousins. Andrea goes there on her own, time to time; I love her for that. I told the story to all of them of what I said to my nieces. So all together, we wished John a "Happy Anniversary."

When someone passes away, we all want some part of him or her to hold on to. I am grateful that John and I had Caitlin together. Because of that, I have a part of him to hold on to. She is a lot like her father in many ways. She has his stubborn streak, his drive, and his "don't mess with me" attitude. I can see him in her every day. I predict that when she becomes an adult, she won't let anything keep her from achieving her goals. I know how proud he would be of her, because I know how proud I will be. She makes me proud every day.

This past year has been a whirlwind of feelings and emotions. Some of the feelings will never go away and I wouldn't want them to. Others have faded some; time really does heal all wounds. I feel whole again and I'm happy with my new life. My hope is that if you are reading this because you needed help in your own grieving process, I have helped you. What you have gone through won't define who you are, but it will make you stronger. Writing all of this has made me stronger and has provided me with the greatest gift. Someday, Caitlin will read this to her own children and they will know that their grandfather was the *"bravest man"* she ever knew.

www.ingramcontent.com/pod-product-compliance
Lightning Source LLC
Chambersburg PA
CBHW020406290526
45785CB00005B/2451